Renal Diet Recipes

Easy and Delicious Recipes to Managing
Kidney Disease, Avoiding Dialysis and
Finally Boost Your Health

Edward Stevens

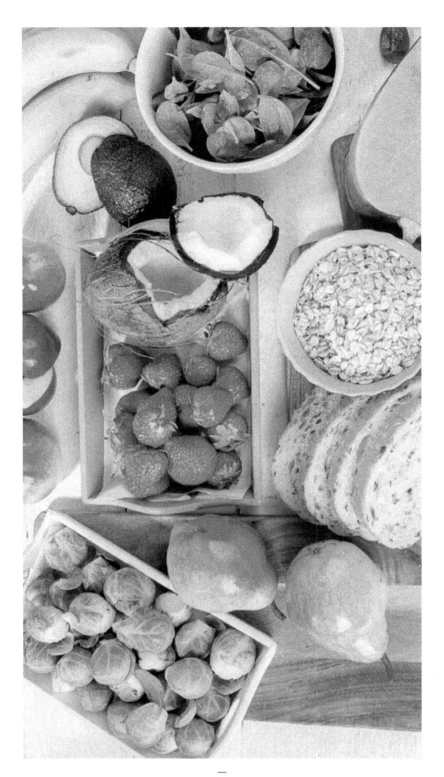

Table of Content

The information in the following pages is broadly considered a truthful and accurate account of facts and as such, any inattention, use, or misuse of the information in question by the reader will render any resulting actions solely under their purview. There are no scenarios in which the publisher or the original author of this work can be in any fashion deemed liable for any hardship or damages that may befall them after undertaking information described herein.

Additionally, the information in the following pages is intended only for informational purposes and should thus be thought of as universal. As befitting its nature, it is presented without assurance regarding its prolonged validity or interim quality. Trademarks that are mentioned are done without written consent and can in no way be considered an endorsement from the trademark holder.

Introduction

Human health hangs in a complete balance when all of its interconnected bodily mechanisms function properly in perfect sync. Without its major organs working normally, the body soon suffers indelible damage. Kidney malfunction is one such example, and it is not just the entire water balance that is disturbed by the kidney disease, but a number of other diseases also emerge due to this problem.

Kidney diseases are progressive, meaning that they can ultimately lead to permanent kidney damage if left unchecked and uncontrolled. That is why it is essential to control and manage the disease and halt its progress, which can be done through medicinal and natural means. While medicines can guarantee only thirty percent of the cure, a change of lifestyle and diet can prove miraculous with their seventy percent guaranteed results. A kidney-friendly diet and lifestyle not only saves the kidneys from excess minerals, but it also aids medicines to work actively. Treatment without a good diet, hence, proves to be useless. In this renal diet cookbook, we shall bring out the basic facts about kidney diseases, their symptoms, causes, and diagnosis. This preliminary introduction can help the readers understand the problem clearly; then, we shall discuss the role of renal diet and kidney-friendly lifestyle in curbing the diseases. It's not just that the book also contains a range of delicious renal diet recipes, which will guarantee luscious flavors and good health.

Despite their tiny size, the kidneys perform a number of functions, which are vital for the body to be able to function healthily.

These include:

- Filtering excess fluids and waste from the blood.

- Creating the enzyme known as renin, which regulates blood pressure.

- Ensuring bone marrow creates red blood cells.

- Controlling calcium and phosphorus levels through absorption and excretion.

Unfortunately, when kidney disease reaches a chronic stage, these functions start to stop working. However, with the right treatment and lifestyle, it is possible to manage symptoms and continue living well. This is even more applicable in the earlier stages of the disease. Tactlessly, 10% of all adults over the age of 20 will experience some form of kidney disease in their lifetime. There are a variety of different treatments for kidney disease, which depend on the cause of the disease.

According to international stats, kidney (or renal) diseases are affecting around 14% of the adult population. In the US, approx. 661.000 Americans suffer from kidney dysfunction. Out of these patients, 468.000 proceed to dialysis treatment, and the rest have one active kidney transplant.

The high quantities of diabetes and heart illness are also related to kidney dysfunction, and sometimes one condition, for example, diabetes, may prompt the other.

With such a significant number of high rates, possibly the best course of treatment is the contravention of dialysis, making people depend upon clinical and crisis facility meds in any occasion multiple times every week. In this manner, if your kidney has just given a few indications of brokenness, you can forestall dialysis through an eating routine, something that we will talk about in this book.

Chapter 1. The Renal Diet

The Benefits of Renal diet

If you have been diagnosed with kidney dysfunction, a proper diet is necessary for controlling the amount of toxic waste in the bloodstream. When toxic waste piles up in the system along with increased fluid, chronic inflammation occurs, and we have a much higher chance of developing cardiovascular, bone, metabolic, or other health issues.

Since your kidneys can't fully get rid of the waste on their own, which comes from food and drinks, probably the only natural way to help our system is through this diet.

A renal diet is especially useful during the first stages of kidney dysfunction and leads to the following benefits:

● Prevents excess fluid and waste build-up

● prevents the progression of renal dysfunction stages

● Decreases the likelihood of developing other chronic health problems, e.g., heart disorders

● has a mild antioxidant function in the body, which keeps inflammation and inflammatory responses under control.

The benefits mentioned above are noticeable once the patient follows the diet for at least a month and then continuing it for longer periods to avoid the stage where dialysis is needed. The diet's strictness depends on the current stage of renal/kidney disease if, for example, if you are in the 3rd or 4th stage, you should follow a stricter diet and be attentive to the food, which is allowed or prohibited.

Nutrients You Need

Potassium

Potassium is a naturally occurring mineral found in nearly all foods in varying amounts. Our bodies need an amount of potassium to help with muscle activity as well as electrolyte balance and regulation of blood pressure. However, if potassium is in excess within the system and the kidneys can't expel it (due to renal disease), fluid retention and muscle spasms can occur.

Phosphorus

Phosphorus is a trace mineral found in a wide range of foods and especially dairy, meat, and eggs. It acts synergistically with calcium as well as Vitamin D to promote bone health. However, when there is damage in the kidneys, excess amounts of the mineral cannot be taken out, causing bone weakness.

Calories

When being on a renal diet, it is vital to give yourself the right number of calories to fuel your system. The exact number of calories you should consume daily depends on your age, gender, general health status, and stage of renal disease. In most cases, though, there are no strict limitations in the calorie intake, as long as you take them from proper sources that are low in sodium, potassium, and phosphorus. In general, doctors recommend a daily limit between 1800-2100 calories per day to keep weight within the normal range.

Protein

Protein is an essential nutrient that our systems need to develop and generate new connective tissue, e.g., muscles, even during injuries. Protein also helps stop bleeding and supports the immune system to fight infections. A healthy adult with no kidney disease would usually need 40-65 grams of protein per day.

However, in a renal diet, protein consumption is a tricky subject as too much or too little can cause problems. When metabolized by our systems, protein also creates waste, which is typically processed by the kidneys. However, when kidneys are damaged or underperforming, as in the case of kidney disease, that waste will stay in the system. This is why patients in more advanced CKD stages are advised to limit their protein consumption as well.

Fats

Our systems need fats and particularly good fats as a fuel source and for other metabolic cell functions. A diet high in bad or trans fats can significantly increase the chances of developing heart problems, which often occur with kidney disease. This is why most physicians advise their renal patients to follow a diet that contains a decent amount of good fats and a meager amount of Trans (processed) or saturated fat.

Sodium

Sodium is what our bodies need to regulate fluid and electrolyte balance. It also plays a role in normal cell division in the muscles and nervous system. However, in kidney disease, sodium can quickly spike at higher than normal levels, and the kidneys will be unable to expel it, causing fluid accumulation as a side-effect. Those who also suffer from heart problems as well should limit its consumption as it may raise blood pressure.

Carbohydrates

Carbs act as a major and quick fuel source for the body's cells. When we consume carbs, our systems turn them into glucose and then into energy for "feeding" our body cells. Carbs are generally not restricted in the renal diet. Still, some types of carbs contain dietary fiber as well, which helps regulate normal colon function and protect blood vessels from damage.

Dietary Fiber

Fiber is an important element in our system that cannot be properly digested, but plays a key role in the regulation of our bowel movements and blood cell protection. The fiber in the renal diet is generally encouraged as it helps loosen up the stools, relieve constipation and bloating and protect from colon damage. However, many patients don't get enough amounts of dietary fiber per day, as many of them are high in potassium or phosphorus. Fortunately, there are some good dietary fiber sources for CKD patients that have lower amounts of these minerals compared to others.

Vitamins/Minerals

According to medical research, our systems need at least 13 vitamins and minerals to keep our cells fully active and healthy. However, patients with renal disease are more likely to be depleted by water-soluble vitamins like B-complex and Vitamin C as a result of limited fluid consumption. Therefore, supplementation with these vitamins, along with a renal diet program, should help cover any possible vitamin deficiencies. Supplementation of fat-soluble vitamins like vitamins A, K, and E may be avoided as they can quickly build up in the system and turn toxic.

Fluids

When you are in an advanced stage of renal disease, fluid can quickly build-up and lead to problems. While it is important to keep your system well hydrated, you should avoid minerals like potassium and sodium, which can trigger further fluid build-up and cause a host of other symptoms.

Nutrient You Need to Avoid

Salt or sodium is known for being one of the most important ingredients that the renal diet prohibits its use. This ingredient, although simple, can badly and strongly affect your body, especially the kidneys. Any excess of sodium can't be easily filtered because of the failing condition of the kidneys. A large build-up of sodium can cause catastrophic results on your body. Potassium and Phosphorus are also prohibited for kidney patients depending on the stage of kidney disease.

Chapter 2. Kidney disease

What is Kidney Disease?

A kidney disease diagnosis implies that the kidneys are either dysfunctional, under-functioning, or damaged and cannot filter out toxins and metabolic waste on their own. Our systems need our kidneys for a waste filtering process. However, when kidney damage occurs, the system is piled up with damaging waste that cannot expel through other means. As a result, inflammatory responses emerge, and you have a much higher chance of developing chronic and serious health disorders like diabetes or heart failure, which can even be fatal in extreme cases.

There are two main types of kidney disease, based on their cause and time duration:

• A sudden and unexpected kidney damage/acute kidney injury (AKI) as a result of an accident or surgery side effects, which usually lasts for a short period of time.

• Chronic and progressive kidney dysfunction (CKD). As its name suggests, this is a chronic condition with multiple progressive stages that lead ultimately to permanent kidney damage. There are approx. 5 stages of the disorder, and during the last and final stage, the patient will need dialysis or a kidney transplant to survive. This final stage is also known in the medical glossary as End-Stage-Renal Disease (ESRD).

There are higher than normal amounts of a certain protein called Arbutin in the urine during all kidney dysfunction stages, which can be confirmed by urine tests for diagnosing renal disease. This condition is known scientifically as Proteinuria. Doctors may also perform blood tests and/or image screening tests to pinpoint a problem with the kidneys and develop a diagnosis.

Causes of Kidney Disease?

There are many causes of kidney disease, including physical injury or disorders that can damage the kidneys, but the two leading causes of kidney disease are diabetes and high blood pressure. These underlying conditions also put people at risk for developing cardiovascular disease. Early treatment may not only slow down the progression of the disease, but also reduce your risk of developing heart disease or stroke.

Kidney disease can affect anyone at any age. African Americans, Hispanics, and American Indians are at increased risk for kidney failure because these groups have a greater prevalence of diabetes and high blood pressure.

Uncontrolled diabetes is the leading cause of kidney disease. Diabetes can damage the kidneys and cause them to fail.

The second leading cause of kidney disease is high blood pressure, also known as hypertension. One in three Americans is at risk for kidney disease because of hypertension. Although there is no cure for hypertension, certain medications, a low-sodium diet, and physical activity can lower blood pressure.

The kidneys help manage blood pressure, but when blood pressure is high, the heart has to work overtime at pumping blood. High blood pressure can damage the blood vessels in the kidneys, reducing their ability to work efficiently. When the force of blood flow is high, blood vessels start to stretch so the blood can flow more easily. The stretching and scarring weaken the blood vessels throughout the entire body, including the kidneys. When the kidneys' blood vessels are injured, they may not remove the waste and extra fluid from the body, creating a dangerous cycle because the extra fluid in the blood vessels can increase blood pressure even more.

Cardiovascular disease is the leading cause of death in the United States. When kidney disease occurs, that process can be affected, and the risk of developing heart disease becomes greater. Cardiovascular disease is an umbrella term used to describe conditions that may damage the heart and blood vessels, including coronary artery disease, heart attack, heart failure, atherosclerosis, and high blood pressure. Complications from a renal disease may develop and can lead to heart disease.

With diabetes, excess blood sugar remains in the bloodstream. The high blood sugar levels can damage the blood vessels in the kidneys and elsewhere in the body. And since high blood pressure is a complication from diabetes, the extra pressure can weaken the walls of the blood vessels, which can lead to a heart attack or stroke.

Other conditions, such as drug abuse and certain autoimmune diseases, can also cause injury to the kidneys. In fact, every drug we put into our body has to pass through the kidneys for filtration. If the drug is not taken following a healthcare provider's instructions, or if it is an illegal substance such as heroin, cocaine, or ecstasy, it can cause injury to the kidneys by raising the blood pressure, also increasing the risk of a stroke, heart failure, and even death.

An autoimmune disease is one in which the immune system, designed to protect the body from illness, sees the body as an invader and attacks its own systems, including the kidneys. Some forms of lupus, for example, attack the kidneys. Another autoimmune disease that can lead to kidney failure is Goodpasture syndrome, a group of conditions that affect the kidneys and the lungs. The damage to the kidneys from autoimmune diseases can lead to chronic kidney disease and kidney failure.

Symptoms of Kidney Disease?

Some people in the early stages of kidney disease may not even show any symptoms. If you suffer from diabetes or high blood pressure, it is important to manage it early on in order to protect your kidneys. Although kidney failure occurs over the course of many years, you may not show any signs until kidney disease or failure has occurred.

When the kidneys are damaged, wastes and toxins can build up in the body because the kidneys cannot filter them as effectively. Once this buildup begins, you may start to feel sick and experience some of the following symptoms:

- Anemia (low red blood cell count)
- Blood in urine
- Bone pain
- Difficulty concentrating
- Difficulty sleeping
- Dry and itchy skin
- Muscle cramps (especially in the legs)
- Nausea
- Poor appetite
- Swelling in feet and ankles
- Tiredness
- Weakness
- Weight loss

Fortunately, once treatment for kidney disease begins, especially if caught in the early stages, symptoms tend to lessen, and general health will begin to improve.

Diagnosis Tests

Besides identifying the symptoms of kidney disease, there are other better and more accurate ways to confirm the extent of loss of renal function. There are mainly two important diagnostic tests:

1. Urine Test

The urine test clearly states all the renal problems. The urine is the waste product of the kidney. When there is a loss of filtration or any hindrance to the kidneys, the urine sample will indicate it through the number of excretory products present in it. The severe stages of chronic disease show some amount of protein and blood in the urine. Do not rely on self-tests; visit an authentic clinic for these tests.

2. Blood Pressure and Blood Test

Another good way to check for renal disease is to test the blood and its composition. A high amount of creatinine and other waste products in the blood clearly indicates that the kidneys are not functioning properly. Blood pressure can also be indicative of renal disease. When the water balance in the body is disturbed, it may cause high blood pressure. Hypertension can both be the cause and symptom of kidney disease and, therefore, should be taken seriously.

Treatment

The best way to manage CKD is to be an active participant in your treatment program, regardless of your stage of renal disease. Proper treatment involves a combination of working with a healthcare team, adhering to a renal diet, and making healthy lifestyle decisions. These can all have a profoundly positive effect on your kidney disease—especially watching how you eat.

Working with Your Healthcare Team

When you have kidney disease, working in partnership with your healthcare team can be extremely important in your treatment program as well as being personally empowering. Regularly meeting with your physician or healthcare team can arm you with resources and information that help you make informed decisions regarding your treatment needs and provide you with a much-needed opportunity to vent, share information, get advice, and receive support in effectively managing this illness.

Adhering to a Renal Diet

The heart of this book is the renal diet. Sticking to this diet can make a huge difference in your health and vitality. Like any change, following the diet may not be easy at first. Important changes to your diet, particularly early on, can possibly prevent the need for dialysis. These changes include limiting salt, eating a low-protein diet, reducing fat intake, and getting enough calories if you need to lose weight. Be honest with yourself first and foremost—learn what you need, and consider your personal goals and obstacles. Start by making small changes. It is okay to have some slip-ups—we all do. With guidance and support, these small changes will become habits of your promising new lifestyle. In no time, you will begin taking control of your diet and health.

Making Healthy Lifestyle Decisions

Lifestyle choices play a crucial part in our health, especially when it comes to helping regulate kidney disease. Lifestyle choices such as allotting time for physical activity, getting enough sleep, managing weight, reducing stress, and limiting smoking and alcohol will help you take control of your overall health, making it easier to manage your kidney disease. Follow this simple formula: Keep toxins out of your body as much as you can, and build up your immune system with a good balance of exercise, relaxation, and sleep.

Chapter 3. BREAKFAST

1. Breakfast Salad from Grains and Fruits

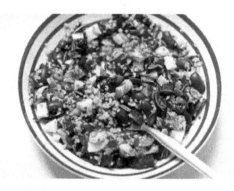

Preparation time: 5 minutes

Cooking time: 15 minutes

Servings: 6

Ingredients:

- 1 8-oz of low-fat vanilla yogurt
- 1 cup of raisins
- 1 orange
- 1 delicious red apple
- 1 Granny Smith apple
- ¾ cup of bulgur
- ¾ cup of quick-cooking brown rice
- ¼ teaspoon of salt
- 3 cups of water

Direction:

1. On high fire, place a large pot and bring water to a boil.

2. Add bulgur and rice. Lower fire to a simmer and cooks for ten minutes while covered.

3. Turn off fire, set aside for 2 minutes while covered.

4. On a baking sheet, transfer and evenly spread grains to cool.

5. Meanwhile, peel oranges and cut them into sections. Chop and core apples.

6. Once grains are cool, transfer to a large serving bowl along with fruits.

7. Add yogurt and mix well to coat.

8. Serve and enjoy.

Nutrition:

- Calories: 187
- Carbs: 4g
- Protein: 8g
- Fats: 3g
- Phosphorus: 45mg
- Potassium: 36mg
- Sodium: 117mg

2. French Toast with Applesauce

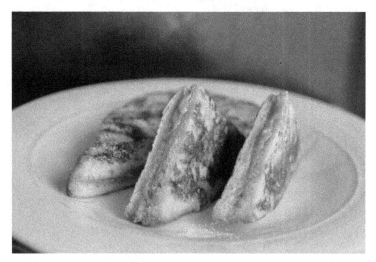

Preparation time: 5 minutes

Cooking time: 15 minutes

Servings: 6

Ingredients:

- ¼ cup of unsweetened applesauce
- ½ cup of milk
- 1 teaspoon of ground cinnamon
- 2 eggs
- 2 tablespoon of white sugar
- 6 slices of whole wheat bread

Directions:

1. Mix well applesauce, sugar, cinnamon, milk, and eggs in a mixing bowl.
2. Dip the bread into applesauce mixture until wet; take note that you should do this one slice at a time.
3. On medium fire, heat a nonstick skillet greased with cooking spray.

4. Add soaked bread one at a time and cook for 2-3 minutes per side or until lightly browned.

5. Serve and enjoy.

Nutrition:

- Calories: 57
- Carbs: 6g
- Protein: 4g
- Fats: 4g
- Phosphorus: 69mg
- Potassium: 88mg
- Sodium: 43mg

3. Bagels Made Healthy

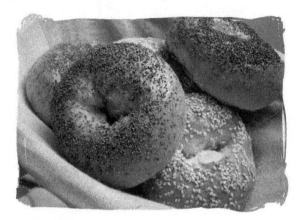

Preparation time: 5 minutes

Cooking time: 25 minutes

Servings: 8

Ingredients:

- 2 teaspoon of yeast
- 1 ½ tablespoon of olive oil
- 1 ¼ cups of bread flour
- 2 cups of whole wheat flour
- 1 tablespoon of vinegar
- 2 tablespoon of honey
- 1 ½ cups of warm water

Directions:

1. In a bread machine, mix all the ingredients, and then process on dough cycle.
2. Once done or end of the cycle, create 8 pieces shaped like a flattened ball.
3. Using your thumb, you must create a hole at the center of each, and then create a donut shape.

4. Place the donut-shaped dough on a greased baking sheet, then covers and let it rise about ½ hour.

5. Prepare about 2 inches of water to boil in a large pan.

6. In boiling water, drop one at a time the bagels and boil for 1 minute, then turn them once.

7. Remove them and return them to a baking sheet and bake at 350oF (175oC) for about 20 to 25 minutes until golden brown.

Nutrition:

- Calories: 221
- Carbs: 42g
- Protein: 7g
- Fats: 3g
- Phosphorus: 130mg
- Potassium: 166mg
- Sodium: 47mg

4. Cornbread with Southern Twist

Preparation time: 15 minutes

Cooking time: 60 minutes

Servings: 8

Ingredients:

- 2 tablespoons of shortening
- 1 ¼ cups of skim milk
- ¼ cup of egg substitute
- 4 tablespoons of sodium-free baking powder
- ½ cup of flour
- 1 ½ cups of cornmeal

Directions:

1. Prepare an 8x8-inch baking dish or a black iron skillet, and then add shortening.
2. Put the baking dish or skillet inside the oven at 425 °F; once the shortening has melted, that means the pan is hot already.
3. In a bowl, add milk and egg, and then mix well.
4. Take out the skillet, and add the melted shortening into the batter and stir well.
5. Pour mixture into skillet after mixing all the ingredients.
6. Cook the cornbread for 15-20 minutes until it is golden brown.

Nutrition:

- Calories: 166
- Carbs: 35g
- Protein: 5g
- Fats: 1g
- Phosphorus: 79mg

- Potassium: 122mg
- Sodium: 34mg

5. Grandma's Pancake Special

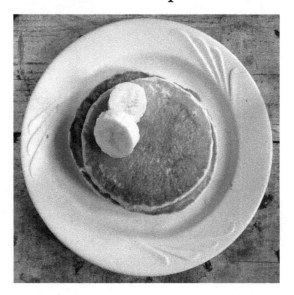

Preparation time: 5 minutes

Cooking time: 15 minutes

Servings: 3

Ingredients:

- 1 tablespoon of oil
- 1 cup of milk
- 1 egg
- 2 teaspoons of sodium-free baking powder
- 2 tablespoons of sugar
- 1 ¼ cups of flour

Directions:

1. Mix together all the dry ingredients, such as the flour, sugar, and baking powder.

2. Combine oil, milk, and egg in another bowl. Once done, add them all to the flour mixture.

3. Make sure that as you stir the mixture; blend them together until slightly lumpy.
4. In a hot, greased griddle, pour-in at least ¼ cup of the batter to make each pancake.
5. To cook, ensure that the bottom is a bit brown, then turn and cook the other side as well.

Nutrition:

- Calories: 167
- Carbs: 50g
- Protein: 11g
- Fats: 11g
- Phosphorus: 176mg
- Potassium: 215mg
- Sodium: 70mg

6. Very Berry Smoothie

Preparation time: 3 minutes

Cooking time: 5 minutes

Servings: 2

Ingredients:

- 2 quarts of water
- 2 cups of pomegranate seeds
- 1 cup of blackberries
- 1 cup of blueberries

Directions:

1. Mix all the ingredients in a blender.
2. Puree until smooth and creamy.
3. Transfer to a serving glass and enjoy.

Nutrition:

- Calories: 464
- Carbs: 111g
- Protein: 8g
- Fats: 4g
- Phosphorus: 132mg
- Potassium: 843mg
- Sodium: 16mg

7. Pasta with Indian Lentils

Preparation time: 5 minutes

Cooking time: 0 minutes

Servings: 6

Ingredients:

- ¼-½ cup of fresh cilantro (chopped)
- 3 cups of water
- 2 small dry red peppers (whole)
- 1 teaspoon of turmeric
- 1 teaspoon of ground cumin
- 2-3 cloves garlic (minced)
- 1 can of diced tomatoes (w/juice)
- 1 large onion (chopped)
- ½ cup of dry lentils (rinsed)
- ½ cup of orzo or tiny pasta

Directions:

1. Combine all the ingredients in the skillet except for the cilantro, and then boil on medium-high heat.
2. Ensure to cover and slightly reduce heat to medium-low and simmer until pasta is tender for about 35 minutes.
3. Afterwards, take out the chili peppers, then add cilantro and top it with low-fat sour cream.

Nutrition:

- Calories: 175
- Carbs: 40g
- Protein: 3g
- Fats: 2g

- Phosphorus: 139mg
- Potassium: 513mg
- Sodium: 61mg

8. Apple Pumpkin Muffins

Preparation Time: 15 minutes

Cooking Time: 20 minutes

Servings: 12

Ingredients:

- 1 cup of all-purpose flour
- 1 cup of wheat bran
- 2 teaspoons of Phosphorus Powder
- 1 cup of pumpkin purée
- ¼ cup of honey
- ¼ cup of olive oil
- 1 egg
- 1 teaspoon of vanilla extract
- ½ cup of cored diced apple

Directions:

1. Preheat the oven to 400°F.
2. Line 12 muffin cups with paper liners.
3. Stir together the flour, wheat bran, and baking powder, mix this in a medium bowl.
4. In a small bowl, whisk together the pumpkin, honey, olive oil, egg, and vanilla.
5. Stir the pumpkin mixture into the flour mixture until just combined.
6. Stir in the diced apple.
7. Spoon the batter in the muffin cups.
8. Bake for about 20 minutes, or until a toothpick inserted in the center of a muffin comes out clean.

Nutrition:

- Calories: 125
- Total Fat: 5g
- Saturated Fat: 1g
- Cholesterol: 18mg
- Sodium: 8mg
- Carbohydrates: 20g
- Fiber: 3g

9. Spiced French Toast

Preparation time: 15 minutes

Cooking time: 12 minutes

Servings: 4

Ingredients:

- 4 eggs
- ½ cup of Homemade Rice Milk (here, or use unsweetened store-bought) or almond milk
- ¼ cup of freshly squeezed orange juice
- 1 teaspoon of ground cinnamon
- ½ teaspoon of ground ginger
- Pinch ground cloves
- 1 tablespoon of unsalted butter, divided
- 8 slices of white bread

Directions

1. Whisk eggs, rice milk, orange juice, cinnamon, ginger, and cloves until well blended in a large bowl.
2. Melt half the butter in a large skillet. It should be in medium-high heat only.
3. Dredge four of the bread slices in the egg mixture until well soaked, and place them in the skillet.
4. Cook the toast until golden brown on both sides, turning once, about 6 minutes total.
5. Repeat with the remaining butter and bread.
6. Serve 2 pieces of hot French toast to each person.

Nutrition:

- Calories: 236

- Total fat: 11g
- Saturated fat: 4g
- Cholesterol: 220mg
- Sodium: 84mg
- Carbohydrates: 27g

10.Breakfast Tacos

Preparation Time: 10 minutes

Cooking Time: 10 minutes

Servings: 4

Ingredients

- 1 teaspoon olive oil
- ½ sweet onion, chopped
- ½ red bell pepper, chopped
- ½ teaspoon minced garlic
- 4 eggs, beaten
- ½ teaspoon ground cumin
- Pinch red pepper flakes
- 4 tortillas
- ¼ cup tomato salsa

Directions:

1. Heat the oil in a large skillet in medium heat only.
2. Add the onion, bell pepper, and garlic, and sauté until softened, about 5 minutes.
3. Add the eggs, cumin, and red pepper flakes, and scramble the eggs with the vegetables until cooked through and fluffy.
4. Spoon 1/4 of the egg mixture into the center of each tortilla, and top each with 1 tablespoon of salsa.
5. Serve immediately.

Nutrition:

- Calories: 211
- Total fat: 7g
- Saturated fat: 2g

- Cholesterol: 211mg

- Sodium: 346mg

- Carbohydrates: 17g

11. Mexican Scrambled Eggs in Tortilla

Preparation Time: 5 minutes

Cooking Time: 2 minutes

Servings: 2

Ingredients:

- 2 medium corn tortillas
- 4 egg whites
- 1 teaspoon of cumin
- 3 teaspoons of green chilies, diced
- ½ teaspoon of hot pepper sauce
- 2 tablespoons of salsa
- ½ teaspoon of salt

Directions

1. Spray some cooking spray on a medium skillet and heat for a few seconds.
2. Whisk the eggs with the green chilies, hot sauce, and comminute
3. Add the eggs into the pan, and whisk with a spatula to scramble. Add the salt.
4. Cook until fluffy and done (1-2 minutes) over low heat.
5. Open the tortillas and spread 1 tablespoon of salsa on each.
6. Distribute the egg mixture onto the tortillas and wrap gently to make a burrito.
7. Serve warm.

Nutrition:

- Calories: 44.1 kcal
- Carbohydrate: 2.23 g
- Protein: 7.69 g

- Sodium: 854 mg
- Potassium: 189 mg

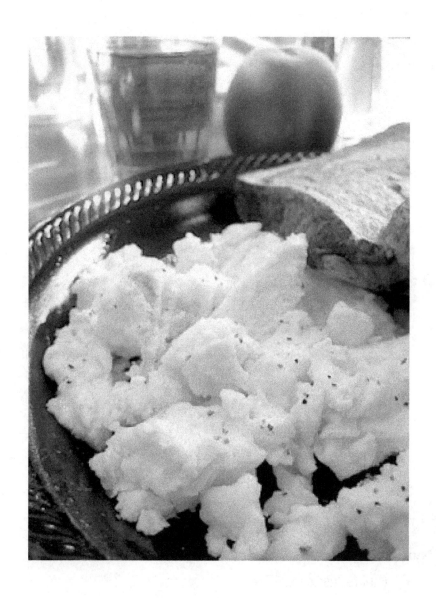

12.American Blueberry Pancakes

Preparation Time: 5 minutes

Cooking Time: 10 minutes

Servings: 6

Ingredients:

- 1 ½ cups of all-purpose flour, sifted
- 1 cup of buttermilk
- 3 tablespoons of sugar
- 2 tablespoons of unsalted butter, melted
- 2 teaspoon of baking powder
- 2 eggs, beaten
- 1 cup of canned blueberries, rinsed

Directions:

1. Combine the baking powder, flour, and sugar in a bowl.
2. Make a hole in the center and slowly add the rest of the ingredients.
3. Begin to stir gently from the sides to the center with a spatula until you get a smooth and creamy batter.
4. With cooking spray, spray the pan and place over medium heat.
5. Take one measuring cup and fill 1/3rd of its capacity with the batter to make each pancake.
6. Use a spoon to pour the pancake batter and let cook until golden brown. Flip once to cook the other side.
7. Serve warm with optional agave syrup.

Nutrition:

- Calories: 251.69 kcal
- Carbohydrate: 41.68 g
- Protein: 7.2 g

- Sodium: 186.68 mg
- Potassium: 142.87 mg
- Phosphorus: 255.39 mg
- Dietary Fiber: 1.9 g

13. Appealing Green Salad

Preparation Time: 50 minutes

Cooking Time: 15 minutes

Serving: 4

Ingredients:

- 1 tbsp. of shallot, minced
- 1/3 cup of olive oil
- 2 tbsp. of fresh lemon juice
- 1 tsp. of honey
- Freshly ground black pepper, to taste

For Salad:

- 1½ cups of chopped broccoli florets
- 1½ cups of shredded cabbage
- 4 cups of chopped lettuce

Directions:

1. In a bowl, add all dressing ingredients and beat until well combined. Keep aside. In another large bowl, mix all salad ingredients.
2. Add dressing and gently toss to coat well. Serve immediately.

Nutrition:

- Calories: 179
- Fat: 17.1g
- Carbs: 7.5g
- Protein: 1.7g
- Fiber: 1.9g
- Potassium: 249mg
- Sodium: 21mg

14. Excellent Veggie Sandwiches

Preparation Time: 30 minutes

Cooking Time: 15 minutes

Serving: 8

Ingredients:

- 1 large sliced tomato
- ½ of sliced cucumber
- ½ cup of thinly sliced red onion
- 1 cup of chopped romaine lettuce leaves
- ½ cup of low-sodium mayonnaise
- 8 toasted white bread slices

Directions:

1. In a large bowl, mix together tomato, cucumber, onion, and lettuce. Spread mayonnaise over each slice evenly.
2. Divide tomato mixture over 4 slices evenly. Cover with remaining slices.
3. With a knife, carefully cut the sandwiches diagonally and serve.

Nutrition:

- Calories: 92
- Fat: 5.3g
- Carbs: 10.5g
- Protein: 1.2g
- Fiber: 0.8g
- Potassium: 112mg
- Sodium: 168mg

15. Lunchtime Staple Sandwiches

Preparation Time: 40 minutes

Cooking Time: 15 minutes

Serving: 2

Ingredients:

- 3 tsp. of low-sodium mayonnaise
- 2 toasted white bread slices
- 3 tbsp. of chopped unsalted cooked turkey
- 2 Thin apple slices
- 2 tbsp. of low-fat cheddar cheese
- 1 tsp. of olive oil

Directions:

1. Spread mayonnaise over each slice evenly.
2. Place turkey over 1 slice, followed by apple slices and cheese.
3. Cover with the remaining slice to make a sandwich.
4. Grease a large nonstick frying pan with oil and heat on medium heat.
5. Place the sandwich in the frying pan, and with the back of the spoon, gently press down.
6. Cook for about 1-2 minutes.
7. Carefully, flip the whole sandwich and cook for about 1-2 minutes.
8. Transfer the sandwich to the serving plate.
9. With a knife, carefully cut the sandwich diagonally and serve.

Nutrition:

- Calories: 239
- Fat: 8.5g
- Carbs: 37.2g
- Protein: 7g

- Fiber: 5.6g
- Potassium: 294mg
- Sodium: 169mg

16. Greek Style Pita Rolls

Preparation Time: 20 minutes

Cooking Time: 15 minutes

Serving: 4

Ingredients:

- 2 (6½-inch) pita breads
- 1 tbsp. of low-fat cream cheese
- 1 peeled, cored, and thinly sliced apple
- Olive oil cooking spray, as required
- 1/8 tsp. of ground cinnamon

Directions:

1. Preheat the oven to 400 °F.
2. In a microwave-safe plate, place tortillas and microwave for about 10 seconds to soften.
3. Spread the cream cheese over each tortilla evenly.
4. Arrange apple slices in the center of each tortilla evenly.
5. Roll tortillas to secure the filling.
6. Arrange the tortilla rolls onto a baking sheet in a single layer.
7. Spray the rolls with cooking spray evenly and sprinkle with cinnamon.
8. Bake for about 10 minutes or until the top becomes golden brown.

Nutrition:

- Calories: 129
- Fat: 2.2g
- Carbs: 24.6g

- Protein: 3.3g
- Fiber: 2.1g
- Potassium: 102mg
- Sodium: 176mg

17.Healthier Pita Veggie Rolls

Preparation Time: 30 minutes

Cooking Time: 15 minutes

Serving: 4

Ingredients:

- 1 cup of shredded romaine lettuce
- 1 seeded and chopped red bell pepper
- ½ cup of chopped cucumber
- 1 small seeded and chopped tomato
- 1 small chopped red onion
- 1 finely minced garlic clove
- 1 tbsp. of olive oil
- ½ tbsp. of fresh lemon juice
- Freshly ground black pepper, to taste
- 3 (6½-inch) pita breads

Directions:

1. In a large bowl, add all ingredients except the pita breads and gently toss to coat well.
2. Arrange pita the breads onto serving plates.
3. Place veggie mixture in the center of each pita bread evenly. Roll the pita bread and serve.

Nutrition:

- Calories: 120
- Fat: 2.8g
- Carbs: 20.7g

- Protein: 3.3g
- Fiber: 1.5g
- Potassium: 156mg
- Sodium: 164mg

18. Crunchy Veggie Wraps

Preparation Time: 60 minutes

Cooking Time: 15 minutes

Serving: 4

Ingredients:

- ¾ cup of shredded purple cabbage
- ¾ cup of shredded green cabbage
- ½ cup of peeled and julienned cucumber
- ½ cup of peeled and julienned carrot
- ¼ cup of chopped walnuts
- 2 tbsp. of olive oil
- 1 tbsp. of fresh lemon juice
- Pinch of salt
- Freshly ground black pepper, to taste
- 6 medium butter lettuce leaves

Directions:

1. In a large bowl, add all ingredients except lettuce and toss to coat well.
2. Place the lettuce leaves onto serving plates.
3. Divide the veggie mixture over each leaf evenly. Top with tofu sauce and serve.

Nutrition:

- Calories: 42
- Fat: 3.1g
- Carbs: 2.9g

- Protein: 1.6g
- Fiber: 1.1g
- Potassium: 106mg
- Sodium: 10mg

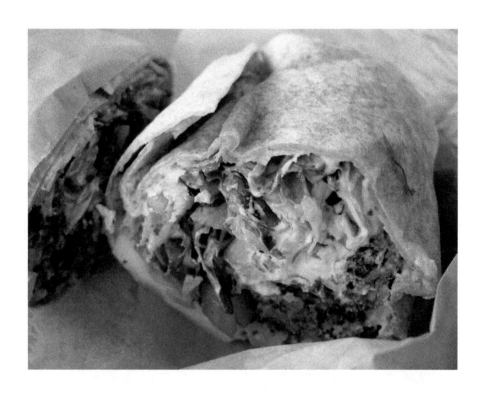

19.Surprisingly Tasty Chicken Wraps

Preparation Time: 50 minutes

Cooking Time: 15 minutes

Serving: 4

Ingredients:

- 4-ounce of cut into strips unsalted cooked chicken breast
- ½ cup of hulled and thinly sliced fresh strawberries
- 1 thinly sliced English cucumber
- 1 tbsp. of chopped fresh mint leaves
- 4 large lettuce leaves

Directions:

1. In a large bowl, add all ingredients except lettuce leaves and gently toss to coat well.
2. Place the lettuce leaves onto serving plates.
3. Divide the chicken mixture over each leaf evenly.
4. Serve immediately.

Nutrition:

- Calories: 74
- Fat: 2.3g
- Carbs: 4.7g
- Protein: 8.9g
- Potassium: 235mg
- Sodium: 27mg

20.   Authentic Shrimp Wraps

Preparation Time: 20 minutes

Cooking Time: 15 minutes

Serving: 4

Ingredients:

- 1 tbsp. of olive oil
- 1 minced garlic clove
- 1 seeded and chopped medium red bell pepper
- ½ pound of peeled, deveined, and chopped medium shrimp
- Pinch of salt
- Freshly ground black pepper, to taste

For Wraps:

- 4 large lettuce leaves

Directions:

1. In a large skillet, heat oil on medium heat.
2. Add garlic and sauté for about 30 seconds.
3. Add bell pepper and cook for about 2-3 minutes.
4. Add shrimp and seasoning and cook for about 2-3 minutes.
5. Remove from heat and cool slightly. Divide shrimp mixture over lettuce leaves evenly. Serve immediately.

Nutrition:

- Calories: 97
- Fat: 4.3g
- Carbs: 3g
- Protein: 12.6g

- Fiber: 0.5g
- Potassium: 81mg
- Sodium: 169mg

21.Loveable Tortillas

Preparation Time: 60 minutes

Cooking Time: 15 minutes

Serving: 4

Ingredients*:*

- ½ cup of low-sodium mayonnaise
- 1 finely minced small garlic clove
- 8-ounce of chopped unsalted cooked chicken
- ½ of seeded and chopped red bell pepper
- ½ of seeded and chopped green bell pepper
- 1 chopped red onion
- 4 (6-ounce) warmed corn tortillas

Directions:

1. In a bowl, mix together mayonnaise and garlic.
2. In another bowl, mix together chicken and vegetables.
3. Arrange the tortillas onto smooth surface.
4. Spread mayonnaise mixture over each tortilla evenly.
5. Place chicken mixture over ¼ of each tortilla.
6. Fold the outside edges inward and roll up like a burrito.
7. Secure each tortilla with toothpicks to secure the filling.
8. Cut each tortilla in half and serve.

Nutrition:

- Calories: 296
- Fat: 8.2g
- Carbs: 44g
- Protein: 13.5g
- Fiber: 5.9g

- Potassium: 262mg
- Sodium: 162mg

22. Cauliflower Rice

Preparation Time: 10 minutes

Cooking Time: 10 minutes

Servings: 4

Ingredients:

- 1 head cauliflower, sliced into florets
- 1 tablespoon of butter
- Black pepper to taste
- 1/4 teaspoon of garlic powder
- 1/4 teaspoon of herb seasoning blend

Direction:

1. Put cauliflower florets in a food processor.
2. Pulse until consistency is similar to grain.
3. In a pan over medium heat, melt the butter and add the spices.
4. Toss cauliflower rice and cook for 10 minutes.
5. Fluff using a fork before serving.

Nutrition:

- Calories: 47
- Protein: 1g
- Carbohydrates: 4g
- Sodium: 43mg
- Potassium: 206mg
- Phosphorus: 31mg
- Calcium: 16mg

23.   Chicken Pineapple Curry

Preparation Time: 40 Minutes

Cooking Time: 3 hours 10 minutes

Servings: 6

Ingredients:

- 1 1/2 lbs. of chicken thighs, boneless, skinless
- 1/2 teaspoon of black pepper
- 1/2 teaspoon of garlic powder
- 2 tablespoons of olive oil
- 20 oz. of canned pineapple
- 2 tablespoons of brown Swerve
- 2 tablespoons of soy sauce
- 1/2 teaspoon of Tabasco sauce
- 2 tablespoons of cornstarch
- 3 tablespoons of water

Direction:

1. Begin by seasoning the chicken thighs with garlic powder and black pepper.
2. Set a suitable skillet over medium-high heat and add the oil to heat.
3. Add the boneless chicken to the skillet and cook for 3 minutes per side.
4. Transfer this seared chicken to a slow cooker, greased with cooking spray.
5. Add 1 cup of the pineapple juice, Swerve, 1 cup of pineapple, tabasco sauce, and soy sauce to a slow cooker.
6. Cover the chicken-pineapple mixture and cook for 3 hours on low heat.

7. Transfer the chicken to the serving plates.

8. Mix the cornstarch with water in a small bowl and pour it into the pineapple curry.

9. Stir and cook this sauce for 2 minutes on high heat until it thickens.

10. Pour this sauce over the chicken and garnish with green onions. Serve warm.

Nutrition:

- Calories: 256
- Fat: 10.4g
- Cholesterol: 67mg
- Sodium: 371mg
- Protein: 22.8g
- Phosphorous: 107mg
- Potassium: 308mg

Chapter 4. Lunch

24.   Baked Pork Chops

Preparation Time: 20 Minutes

Cooking Time: 40minutes

Servings: 6

Ingredients:

- 1/2 cup of flour
- 1 large egg
- 1/4 cup of water
- 3/4 cup of breadcrumbs
- 6 (3 1/2 oz.) of pork chops
- 2 tablespoons of butter, unsalted
- 1 teaspoon of paprika

Direction:

1. Begin by switching the oven to 350 °F to preheat.
2. Mix and spread the flour on a shallow plate.
3. Whisk the egg with water in another shallow bowl.
4. Spread the breadcrumbs on a separate plate.
5. Firstly, coat the pork with flour, then dip in the egg mix and then in the crumbs.
6. Grease a baking sheet and place the chops in it.
7. Drizzle the pepper on top and bake for 40 minutes.
8. Serve.

Nutrition:

- Calories: 221

- Sodium: 135mg

- Carbohydrate: 11.9g

- Protein: 24.7g

- Phosphorous: 299mg

- Potassium: 391mg

25.   Lasagna Rolls in Marinara Sauce

Preparation Time: 15 Minutes

Cooking Time: 30 minutes

Servings: 9

Ingredients:

- ¼ tsp. of crushed red pepper
- ¼ tsp. of salt
- ½ cup of shredded mozzarella cheese
- ½ cups of parmesan cheese, shredded
- 1 14-oz. of package tofu, cubed
- 1 25-oz. of a can of low-sodium marinara sauce
- 1 tbsp. of extra virgin olive oil
- 12 whole of wheat lasagna noodles
- 2 tbsp. of Kalamata olives, chopped
- 3 cloves minced garlic
- 3 cups of spinach, chopped

Directions:

1. Put enough water on a large pot and cook the lasagna noodles according to the package. Drain, rinse, and set aside until ready to use. In a large skillet, sauté garlic over medium heat for 20 seconds. Add the tofu and spinach and cook until the spinach wilts. Transfer this mixture to a bowl and add parmesan olives, salt, red pepper, and 2/3 cup of the marinara sauce.

2. In a pan, spread a cup of marinara sauce on the bottom. To make the rolls, place noodle on a surface and spread ¼ cup of the tofu filling. Roll up and place it on the pan with the marinara sauce. Do this procedure until all lasagna noodles are rolled.

---

3. Place the pan over high heat and bring to a simmer. Reduce the heat to medium and let it cook for three more minutes. Sprinkle mozzarella cheese and let the cheese melt for two minutes. Serve hot.

Nutrition:

- Calories: 600
- Carbs: 65g
- Protein: 36g
- Phosphorus: 627mg
- Potassium: 914mg
- Sodium: 1194mg

26.   Chicken Curry

Preparation Time: 10 Minutes

Cooking Time: 9 Hours

Servings: 5

Ingredients:

- 2 to 3 boneless chicken breasts
- ¼ cup of chopped green onions
- 1 can of 4 oz. of diced green chili peppers
- 2 teaspoons of minced garlic
- 1 and 1/2 teaspoons of curry powder
- 1 teaspoon of chili Powder
- 1 teaspoon of cumin
- ½ teaspoon of cinnamon
- 1 teaspoon of lime juice
- 1 and 1/2 cups of water
- 1 can or 7 oz. of coconut milk
- 2 cups of white cooked rice
- Chopped cilantro, for garnish

Direction:

1. Combine the green onion with the chicken, the green chili peppers, the garlic, the curry powder, the chili powder, the cumin, the cinnamon, the lime juice, and the water in the bottom of a 6-qt slow cooker.

2. Cover the slow cooker with a lid and cook your ingredients on Low for about 7 to 9 hours.

3. After the cooking time ends up, shred the chicken with the help of a fork.

4. Add in the coconut milk and cook on High for about 15 minutes.

5. Top the chicken with cilantro; then serve your dish with rice.

6. Enjoy your lunch!

Nutrition:

- Calories: 254
- Fats: 18g
- Carbs: 6g
- Fiber: 1.6g
- Potassium: 370mg
- Sodium: 240mg
- Phosphorous: 114mg
- Protein 17g

27. Steak with Onion

Preparation Time: 5 Minutes

Cooking Time: 60 Minutes

Servings: 7-8

Ingredients:

- ¼ cup of white flour
- 1/8 Teaspoon of ground black pepper
- 1 and ½ pounds of round steak of ¾ inch of thickness each
- 2 tablespoons of oil
- 1 cup of water
- 1 tablespoon of vinegar
- 1 Minced garlic clove
- 1 to 2 bay leaves
- ¼ teaspoon of crushed dried thyme
- 3 Sliced medium onions

Directions:

1. Cut the steak into about 7 to 8 equal Servings. Combine the flour and the pepper, then pound the Ingredients all together into the meat. Heat the oil in a large skillet over medium-high heat and brown the meat on both its sides.

2. Remove the meat from the skillet and set it aside Combine the water with the vinegar, the garlic, the bay leaf, and the thyme in the skillet; then bring the mixture to a boil.

3. Place the meat in the mixture and cover it with onion slices.

4. Cover your ingredients and let simmer for about 55 to 60 minutes.

5. Serve and enjoy your lunch!

Nutrition:

- Calories: 286
- Fats: 18g
- Carbs: 12g
- Fiber: 2.25g
- Potassium: 368mg
- Sodium: 45mg
- Phosphorous: 180mg
- Protein: 19g

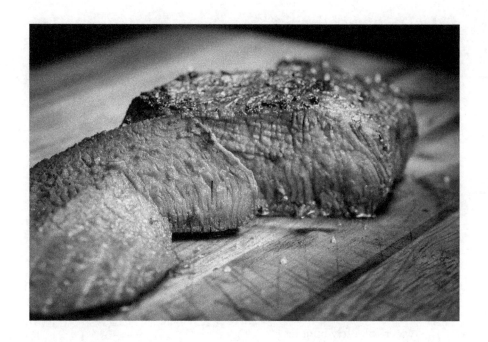

28.   Shrimp Scampi

Preparation Time: 4 Minutes

Cooking Time: 8 Minutes

Servings: 3

Ingredients:

- 1 tablespoon of olive oil
- 1 minced garlic clove
- ½ pound of cleaned and peeled shrimp
- ¼ cup of dry white wine
- 1 tablespoon of lemon juice
- ½ teaspoon of basil
- 1 tablespoon of chopped fresh parsley
- 4 oz. of dry linguini

Directions:

1. Heat the oil in a large non-stick skillet; then add the garlic and the shrimp and cook while stirring for about 4 minutes.
2. Add the wine, the lemon juice, the basil, and the parsley.
3. Cook for about 5 minutes longer; then boil the linguini in unsalted water for a few minutes.
4. Drain the linguini, then top it with the shrimp.
5. Serve and enjoy your lunch!

Nutrition:

- Calories: 340
- Fats: 26g

- Carbs: 11.3g
- Fiber: 2.1g
- Potassium: 189mg
- Sodium: 85mg
- Phosphorous: 167mg
- Protein: 15g

29.   Chicken Paella

Preparation Time: 5 Minutes

Cooking Time: 10 Minutes

Servings: 8

Ingredients:

- ½ pound of skinned, boned, and cut into pieces chicken breasts
- 1/4 cup of water
- 1 can of 10-1/2 oz. of low-sodium chicken broth
- ½ pound of peeled and cleaned medium-size shrimp
- 1/2 cup of frozen green pepper
- 1/3 cup of chopped red bell
- 1/3 cup of thinly sliced green onion
- 2 minced garlic cloves
- 1/4 teaspoon of pepper
- 1 dash of ground saffron
- 1 cup of uncooked instant white rice

Direction:

1. Combine the first 3 ingredients in a medium casserole, cover it with a lid, then microwave it for about 4 minutes.
2. Stir in the shrimp and the following 6 ingredients; then cover and microwave the shrimp on high heat for about 3 and ½ minutes.
3. Stir in the rice, then cover and set aside for about 5 minutes.
4. Serve and enjoy your paella!

Nutrition:

- Calories: 236
- Fats: 11g
- Carbs: 6g

- Fiber: 1.2g
- Potassium: 178mg
- Sodium: 83mg
- Phosphorous: 144mg
- Protein: 28g

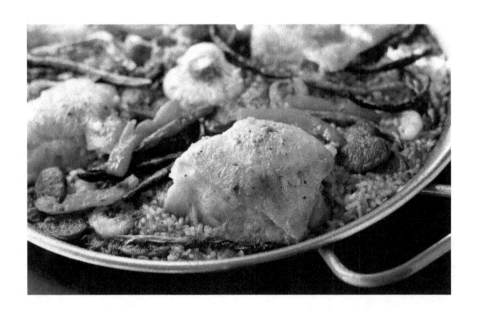

30.   Beef Kabobs with Pepper

Preparation Time: 5 Minutes

Cooking Time: 10 Minutes

Servings: 8

Ingredients:

- 1 Pound of beef sirloin
- ½ cup of vinegar
- 2 tbsp. of salad oil
- 1 medium chopped onion
- 2 tbsp. of chopped fresh parsley
- ¼ tsp. of black pepper
- 2 Cut into strips green peppers

Directions*:*

1. Trim the fat from the meat, then cut it into cubes of 1 and ½ inches each.
2. Mix the vinegar, the oil, the onion, the parsley, and the pepper in a bowl.
3. Place the meat in the marinade and set it aside for about 2 hours; make sure to stir from time to time.
4. Remove the meat from the marinade and alternate it on skewers instead with green pepper.
5. Brush the pepper with the marinade and broil for about 10 minutes 4 inches from the heat.
6. Serve and enjoy your kabobs.

Nutrition:

- Calories: 357
- Fats: 24g
- Carbs: 9g
- Fiber: 2.3g
- Potassium: 250mg
- Sodium: 60mg
- Phosphorous: 217mg
- Protein: 26g

31. Chicken, Corn and Peppers

Preparation Time: 5 minutes

Cooking Time: 1 hour

Servings: 4

Ingredients:

- 2 pounds chicken breast, skinless, boneless, and cubed
- 2 tablespoons of olive oil
- 2 garlic cloves, minced
- 1 red onion, chopped
- 2 red bell peppers, chopped
- ¼ teaspoon of cumin, ground
- 2 cups of corn
- ½ cup of chicken stock
- 1 teaspoon of chili powder
- ¼ cup of cilantro, chopped

Directions:

1. Heat up a pot with the oil over medium-high heat, add the chicken, and brown for 4 minutes on each side.
2. Add the onion and the garlic and sauté for 5 minutes more.
3. Add the rest of the ingredients, stir, bring to a simmer over medium heat, and cook for 45 minutes.
4. Divide into bowls and serve.

Nutrition:

- Calories: 332
- Fat: 16.1
- Fiber: 8.4
- Carbs: 25.4

- Protein: 17.4

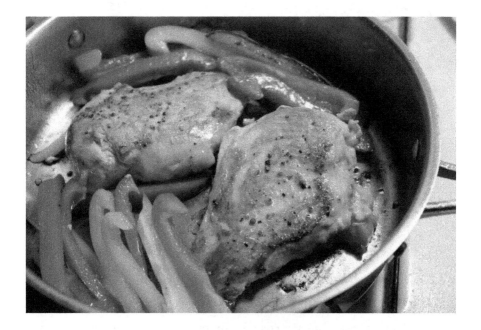

Chapter 5. Dinner

32.   Eggplant and Red Pepper Soup

Preparation Time: 20 minutes

Cooking Time: 40 minutes

Servings: 6

Ingredients:

- 1 small sweet onion, cut into quarters
- 2 small red bell peppers, halved
- 2 cups of cubed eggplant
- 2 cloves garlic, crushed
- 1 tbsp. of olive oil
- 1 cup of chicken stock
- Water
- ¼ cup of chopped fresh basil
- Ground black pepper

Directions:

1. Preheat the oven to 350F.
2. Put the onions, red peppers, eggplant, and garlic in a baking dish.
3. Drizzle the vegetables with the olive oil.
4. Roast the vegetables for 30 minutes or until they are slightly charred and soft.
5. Cool the vegetables slightly and remove the skin from the peppers.
6. Puree the vegetables with a hand mixer (with the chicken stock).
7. Transfer the soup to a medium pot and add enough water to reach the desired thickness.

8. Heat the soup to a simmer and add the basil.

9. Season with pepper and serve.

Nutrition:

- Calories: 61
- Fat: 2g
- Carb: 9g
- Phosphorus: 33mg
- Potassium: 198mg
- Sodium: 98mg
- Protein: 2g

33.   Seafood Casserole

Preparation Time: 20 minutes

Cooking Time: 45 minutes

Servings: 6

Ingredients:

- 2 cups of eggplant peeled and diced into 1-inch pieces
- Butter, for greasing the baking dish
- 1 tbsp. of olive oil
- ½ sweet onion, chopped
- 1 tsp. of minced garlic
- 1 celery stalk, chopped
- ½ red bell pepper, boiled and chopped
- 3 tbsp. of freshly squeezed lemon juice
- 1 tsp. of hot sauce
- ¼ tsp. of Creole seasoning mix
- ½ cup of white rice, uncooked
- 1 large egg
- 4 ounces of cooked shrimp
- 6 ounces of Queen crab meat

Directions:

1. Preheat the oven to 350F. Boil the eggplant in a saucepan for 5 minutes. Drain and set aside.
2. Grease a 9-by-13-inch baking dish with butter and set aside. Heat the olive oil in a large skillet over medium heat.
3. Sauté the garlic, onion, celery, and bell pepper for 4 minutes or until tender

4. Add the sautéed vegetables to the eggplant, along with the lemon juice, hot sauce, seasoning, rice, and egg. Stir to combine. Fold in the shrimp and crab meat.

5. Spoon the casserole mixture into the casserole dish, patting down the top.

6. Bake for 25 to 30 minutes or until casserole is heated through and rice is tender.

7. Serve warm.

Nutrition:

- Calories: 61
- Fat: 2g
- Carb: 9g
- Phosphorus: 23mg
- Potassium: 178mg
- Sodium: 98mg
- Protein: 2g

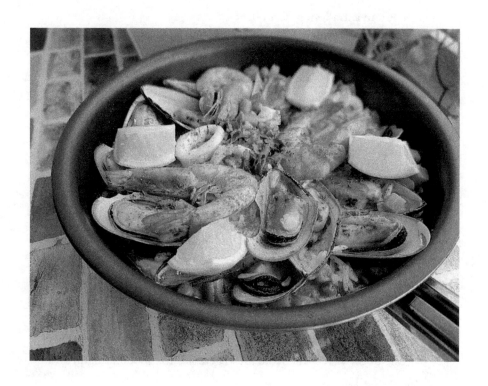

34.   Ground Beef and Rice Soup

Preparation Time: 15 minutes

Cooking Time: 40 minutes

Servings: 6

Ingredients:

- ½ pound extra-lean ground beef
- ½ small sweet onion, chopped
- 1 tsp. of minced garlic
- 2 cups of water
- 1 cup of low-sodium beef broth
- ½ cup of long-grain white rice, uncooked
- 1 celery stalk, chopped
- ½ cup of Fresh green beans, cut into – 1-inch pieces
- 1 tsp. of chopped fresh thyme
- Ground black pepper

Directions:

1. Sauté the ground beef in a saucepan for 6 minutes or until the beef is completely browned. Drain off the excess fat and add the onion and garlic to the saucepan. Sauté the vegetables for about 3 minutes, or until they are softened

2. Add the celery, rice, beef broth, and water. Bring the soup to a boil, reduce the heat to low, and simmer for 30 minutes or until the rice is tender.

3. Add the green beans and thyme and simmer for3 minutes. Remove the soup from the heat and season with pepper.

Nutrition:

- Calories: 51
- Fat: 2g
- Carb: 9g
- Phosphorus: 63mg
- Potassium: 198mg
- Sodium: 128mg
- Protein: 2g

35.   Couscous Burgers

Preparation Time: 20 minutes

Cooking Time: 10 minutes

Servings: 4

Ingredients:

- ½ cup of canned chickpeas, rinsed and drained
- 2 tbsp. of chopped fresh cilantro
- Chopped fresh parsley
- 1 tbsp. of lemon juice
- 2 tsp. of lemon zest
- 1 tsp. of minced garlic
- 2 ½ cups of cooked couscous
- 2 lightly beaten eggs
- 2 tbsp. of olive oil

Directions:

1. Put the cilantro, chickpeas, parsley, lemon juice, lemon zest, and garlic in a food processor and pulse until a paste form.
2. Transfer the chickpea mixture to a bowl and add the eggs and couscous. Mix well.
3. Chill the mixture in the refrigerator for 1 hour.
4. Form the couscous mixture into 4 patties.
5. Heat olive oil in a skillet.
6. Place the patties in the skillet, 2 at a time, gently pressing them down with a spatula.
7. Cook for 5 minutes or until golden and flip the patties over.

8. Cook the other side for 5 minutes and transfer the cooked burgers to a plate covered with a paper towel. Repeat with the remaining 2 burgers.

Nutrition:

- Calories: 61
- Fat: 2g
- Carb: 9g
- Phosphorus: 133mg
- Potassium: 168mg
- Sodium: 108mg
- Protein: 2g

Chapter 6. Desserts

36.   Moo-Less Chocolate Mousse

Preparation Time: 10 minutes

Cooking Time: 5 minutes

Servings: 2

Ingredients:

- 2 ripe avocados
- 1 ripe banana
- 1/4 cup of unsweetened cacao powder
- 2-4 tbsp. of coconut milk
- 1-4 tbsp. of maple syrup
- 1/2 tsp. of pure vanilla extract
- 1 pinch of cinnamon
- 1 pinch of sea salt

Directions:

1. Scoop out the flesh of the avocados and mash by hand.
2. Add all the ingredients to a blender and process until creamy.
3. Serve in 2 bowls. Garnish with toasted hazelnuts.

Nutrition:

- Calories: 346
- Carbs: 35g
- Fat: 26g
- Protein: 6g

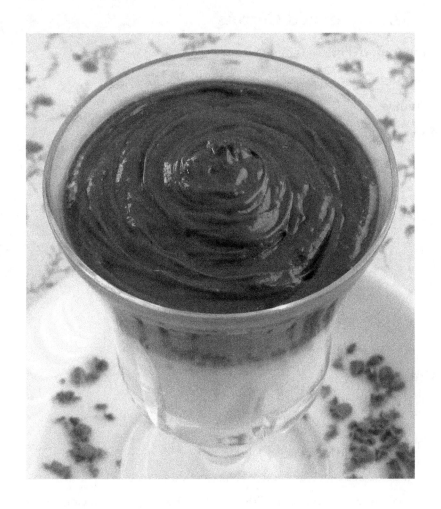

37.   Baked Carrots

Preparation Time: 40 minutes

Cooking Time: 25 minutes

Servings: 3

Ingredients:

- 1 tbsp. of butter
- 3 cloves garlic
- Zest and juice of 1 orange
- Handful of fresh parsley leaves
- 1 lb. of carrots
- ½ cup of extra-virgin olive oil
- 1 cup of chicken stock
- Salt and pepper to taste

Directions:

1. Mince the garlic.
2. Slice the carrots very thinly.
3. Chop the fresh parsley leaves.
4. Mix in a bowl the garlic, orange zest, and parsley.
5. Cover a roasting dish with some butter and put the previous mixture on it.
6. Arrange carrot slices on the bottom, add some olive oil on top, sprinkle with salt, pepper, garlic, zest, and parsley mixture.
7. Repeat the previous step until you go out of carrots.
8. Add orange juice and chicken stock.
9. Cover with a piece of wax paper. Bake for 20-25 minutes until carrots are fork-tender.

Nutrition:

- Calories: 109
- Fat: 5.8g
- Carbs: 14g
- Protein: 1.4g

Chapter 7. Smoothies and Drinks

38. Berry Cucumber Smoothie

Preparation Time: 10minutes

Cooking Time: 0 minutes

Servings: 1

Ingredients:

- 1 medium cucumber, peeled and sliced
- ½ cup of fresh blueberries
- ½ cup of fresh or frozen strawberries
- ½ cup of unsweetened rice milk
- Stevia, to taste

Directions:

1. First, start by putting all the ingredients in a blender jug.
2. Give it a pulse for 30 seconds until blended well.
3. Serve chilled and fresh.

Nutrition:

- Calories: 141
- Protein: 10 g
- Carbohydrates: 15 g
- Fat: 0 g
- Sodium: 113 mg
- Potassium: 230 mg
- Phosphorus: 129 mg

39.   Raspberry Peach Smoothie

Preparation Time: 10 minutes

Cooking Time: 0 minutes

Servings: 2

Ingredients:

- 1 cup of frozen raspberries
- 1 medium peach, pit removed, sliced
- ½ cup of silken tofu
- 1 tbsp. of honey
- 1 cup of unsweetened vanilla almond milk

Directions:

1. First, start by putting all the ingredients in a blender jug.
2. Give it a pulse for 30 seconds until blended well.
3. Serve chilled and fresh.

Nutrition:

- Calories: 132
- Protein: 9g
- Carbohydrates: 14 g
- Sodium: 112 mg
- Potassium: 310 mg
- Phosphorus: 39 mg
- Calcium: 32 mg

40.   Power-Boosting Smoothie

Preparation Time: 5 minutes

Cooking Time: 0 minutes

Servings: 2

Ingredients:

- ½ cup of water
- ½ cup of non-dairy whipped topping
- 2 scoops of whey protein powder
- 1½ cups of frozen blueberries

Directions:

1. In a high-speed blender, add all the ingredients and pulse until smooth.
2. Transfer into 2 serving glass and serve immediately.

Nutrition:

- Calories: 242
- Fat: 7g
- Carbs: 23.8g
- Protein: 23.2g
- Potassium (K): 263mg
- Sodium (Na): 63mg
- Phosphorous: 30 mg

41.Distinctive Pineapple Smoothie

Preparation Time: 5 minutes

Cooking Time: 0 minutes

Servings: 2

Ingredients:

- ¼ cup of crushed ice cubes
- 2 scoops of vanilla whey protein powder
- 1 cup of water
- 1½ cups of pineapple

Directions:

1. In a high-speed blender, add all the ingredients and pulse until smooth.
2. Transfer into 2 serving glass and serve immediately.

Nutrition:

- Calories: 117
- Fat: 2.1g
- Carbs: 18.2g
- Protein: 22.7g
- Potassium (K): 296mg
- Sodium (Na): 81mg
- Phosphorous: 28 mg

Chapter 8. Soups and Stews

42.   Lamb Stew

Preparation Time: 30 minutes

Cooking Time: 1 hour and 40 minutes

Servings: 6

Ingredients:

- 1 lb. boneless lamb shoulder, trimmed and cubes
- Black pepper to taste
- ¼ cup of all-purpose flour
- 1 tablespoon of olive oil
- 1 onion, chopped
- 3 garlic cloves, chopped
- ½ cup tomato sauce
- 2 cups of low-sodium beef broth
- 1 teaspoon of dried thyme
- 2 parsnips, sliced
- 2 carrots, sliced
- 1 cup of frozen peas

Directions:

1. Season the lamb with pepper
2. Coat it evenly with flour.
3. Pour oil in a pot over medium heat.
4. Cook the lamb and then set aside.

5. Add onion to the pot.

6. Cook for 2 minutes.

7. Add garlic and sauté for 30 seconds.

8. Pour in the broth to deglaze the pot.

9. Add the tomato sauce and thyme.

10. Put the lamb back in the pot.

11. Bring to a boil and then simmer for 1 hour.

12. Add parsnips and carrots.

13. Cook for 30 minutes.

14. Add green peas and cook for 5 minutes.

Nutrition:

- Calories: 156
- Total Fat: 11g
- Cholesterol: 26mg
- Carbohydrates: 17g
- Fiber: 3g
- Protein: 7g
- Phosphorus: 115mg
- Potassium: 567mg
- Sodium: 148mg

43.   Sausage & Egg Soup

Preparation Time: 15 minutes

Cooking Time: 30 minutes

Servings: 4

Ingredients:

- ½ lb. ground beef
- Black pepper
- ½ teaspoon of ground sage
- ½ teaspoon of garlic powder
- ½ teaspoon of dried basil
- 4 slices bread (one day old), cubed
- 2 tablespoons of olive oil
- 1 tablespoon of herb seasoning blend
- 2 garlic cloves, minced
- 3 cups of low-sodium chicken broth
- 1 cup of water
- 4 tablespoons of fresh parsley
- 4 eggs
- 2 tablespoons of Parmesan cheese, grated

Directions:

1. Preheat your oven to 375 °F.
2. Mix the first five ingredients to make the sausage. Toss bread cubes in oil and seasoning blend.
3. Bake in the oven for 8 minutes. Set aside.
4. Cook the sausage in a pan over medium heat.

5. Cook the garlic in the sausage drippings for 2 minutes.

6. Stir in the broth, water, and parsley.

7. Bring to a boil and then simmer for 10 minutes.

8. Pour into serving bowls and top with baked bread, egg and sausage.

Nutrition:

- Calories: 196
- Fat: 11g
- Cholesterol: 26mg
- Carbohydrates: 17g
- Fiber: 3g
- Protein: 7g
- Phosphorus: 125mg
- Potassium: 537mg
- Sodium: 148mg

44.   Spring Veggie Soup

Preparation Time: 20 minutes

Cooking Time: 45 minutes

Servings: 5

Ingredients:

- 2 tablespoons of olive oil
- ½ cup of onion, diced
- ½ cup of mushrooms, sliced
- 1/8 cup of celery, chopped
- 1 tomato, diced
- ½ cup of carrots, diced
- 1 cup of green beans, trimmed
- ½ cup of frozen corn
- 1 teaspoon of garlic powder
- 1 teaspoon of dried oregano leaves
- 4 cups of low-sodium vegetable broth

Directions:

1. In a pot, pour the olive oil and cook the onion and celery for 2 minutes.
2. Add the rest of the ingredients.
3. Bring to a boil.
4. Reduce heat and simmer for 45 minutes.

Nutrition:

- Calories: 136

- Total Fat: 11g
- Cholesterol: 26mg
- Carbohydrates: 17g
- Fiber: 3g
- Protein: 7g
- Phosphorus: 125mg
- Potassium: 527mg
- Sodium: 138mg

Chapter 9. Vegetables

45. Braised Carrots 'n Kale

Preparation Time: 10 minutes

Cooking Time: 10 minutes

Servings: 2

Ingredients:

- 1 tablespoon of coconut oil
- 1 onion, sliced thinly
- 5 cloves of garlic, minced
- 3 medium carrots, sliced thinly
- 10 ounces of kale, chopped
- ½ cup of water
- Salt and pepper to taste
- A dash of red pepper flakes

Directions:

1. Heat the oil in a skillet over medium flame and sauté the onion and garlic until fragrant. Toss in the carrots and stir for 1 minute. Add the kale and water. Season it with salt and pepper to taste.
2. Close the lid and allow simmering for 5 minutes.
3. Sprinkle with red pepper flakes.
4. Serve and enjoy.

Nutrition:

- Calories: 161
- Fat: 8g
- Carbs: 20g
- Protein: 8g
- Fiber: 6g
- Sodium: 63mg
- Potassium: 900mg

46.   Butternut Squash Hummus

Preparation Time: 10 minutes

Cooking Time: 15 minutes

Servings: 8

Ingredients:

- 2 pounds butternut squash, seeded and peeled
- 1 tablespoon of olive oil
- ¼ cup of tahini
- 2 tablespoons of lemon juice
- 2 cloves of garlic, minced
- Salt and pepper to taste

Directions:

1. Heat the oven to 300 °F.
2. Coat the butternut squash with olive oil.
3. Place in a baking dish and bake for 15 minutes in the oven.
4. Once the squash is cooked, place it in a food processor together with the rest of the ingredients.
5. Pulse it until smooth.
6. Place in individual containers.
7. Put a label and store it in the fridge.
8. Allow warming at room temperature before heating in the microwave oven.
9. Serve with carrots or celery sticks.

Nutrition:

- Calories: 109
- Fat: 6g
- Carbs: 15g
- Protein: 2g
- Fiber: 4g
- Sodium: 14mg
- Potassium: 379mg

47.   Stir Fried Gingery Veggies

Preparation Time: 10 minutes

Cooking Time: 10 minutes

Servings: 4

Ingredients:

- 1 tablespoon of oil
- 3 cloves of garlic, minced
- 1 onion, chopped
- 1 thumb-size ginger, sliced
- 1 tablespoon of water
- 1 large carrot, peeled and julienned
- 1 large green bell pepper, seeded and julienned
- 1 large yellow bell pepper, seeded and julienned
- 1 large red bell pepper, seeded and julienned
- 1 zucchini, julienned
- Salt and pepper to taste

Directions:

1. Heat oil in a nonstick saucepan over a high flame and sauté the garlic, onion, and ginger until fragrant.
2. Stir in the rest of the ingredients.
3. Keep on stirring for at least 5 minutes until vegetables are tender.
4. Serve and enjoy.

Nutrition:

- Calories: 70

- Fat: 4g
- Carbs: 9g
- Protein: 1g
- Fiber: 2g
- Sodium: 273mg
- Potassium: 263mg
- Vegetables: 2

48.   Cauliflower Fritters

Preparation Time: 10 minutes

Cooking Time: 15 minutes

Servings: 6

Ingredients:

- 1 large cauliflower head, cut into florets
- 2 eggs, beaten
- ½ teaspoon of turmeric
- ½ teaspoon of salt
- ¼ teaspoon of black pepper
- 1 tablespoon of coconut oil

Directions:

1. Place the cauliflower florets in a pot with water and bring to a boil. Cook until tender, around 5 minutes of boiling. Drain well.
2. Place the cauliflower, eggs, turmeric, salt, and pepper into the food processor.
3. Pulse until the mixture becomes coarse.
4. Transfer into a bowl. Using your hands, form six small-flattened balls and place in the fridge for at least 1 hour until the mixture hardens.
5. Heat the oil in a nonstick pan and fry the cauliflower patties for 3 minutes on each side.
6. Serve and enjoy.

Nutrition:

- Calories: 53
- Fat: 6g
- Carbs: 2g
- Protein: 3g
- Fiber: 1g
- Sodium: 228mg
- Potassium: 159mg

49.   Stir-Fried Squash

Preparation Time: 10 minutes

Cooking Time: 10 minutes

Servings: 4

Ingredients:

- 1 tablespoon of olive oil
- 3 cloves of garlic, minced
- 1 butternut squash, seeded and sliced
- 1 tablespoon of coconut aminos
- 1 tablespoon of lemon juice
- 1 tablespoon of water
- Salt and pepper to taste

Directions:

1. Heat the oil over medium flame and sauté the garlic until fragrant.
2. Stir in the squash for another 3 minutes before adding the rest of the ingredients.
3. Close the lid and allow to simmer for 5 more minutes or until the squash is soft.
4. Serve and enjoy.

Nutrition:

- Calories: 83
- Fat: 3g
- Carbs: 14g
- Protein: 2g

50.   Cauliflower Hash Brown

Preparation Time: 10 minutes

Cooking Time: 20 minutes

Servings: 6

Ingredients:

- 4 eggs, beaten
- ½ cup of coconut milk
- ½ teaspoon of dry mustard
- Salt and pepper to taste
- 1 large head cauliflower, shredded

Directions:

1. Place all the ingredients in a mixing bowl and mix until well combined. Place a nonstick fry pan and heat over medium flame.
2. Add a large dollop of cauliflower mixture in the skillet.
3. Fry one side for 3 minutes, flip and cook the other side for a minute, like a pancake. Repeat the process to the remaining ingredients.
4. Serve and enjoy.

Nutrition:

- Calories: 102
- Fat: 8g
- Carbs: 4g
- Protein: 5g
- Fiber: 1g
- Sodium: 63mg

Conclusion

Kidney disease is now ranked as the 18th deadliest disease in the world. In the United States alone, it is estimated that more than 600,000 Americans have kidney failure.

These statistics are concerning, so it is essential that you take proper care of your kidneys, starting with a kidney-friendly diet.

In this e-book, you will learn that management creates healthy, tasty, and kidney-friendly dishes.

These recipes are ideal whether you have been diagnosed with a kidney problem or want to avoid it.

When it comes to your well-being and health, it's a good idea to visit your doctor as often as possible to make sure you don't experience problems that you may not have. The kidneys are your body's channel for toxins (like the liver), cleaning the blood of distant substances and toxins that are flushed out by things like food preservatives and other toxins.

Where you eat fluffy and fill your body with toxins, whether from food, beverages (for example, drink or alcohol) or even the air you breathe (free radicals are in the sun and move through your skin, through dirty air), and many food sources contain them). Your body will generally convert a lot of things that appear to be benign until your body organs convert them to things like formaldehyde due to the synthetic response and metamorphic phase.

An example is a large part of these dietary sugars that are used in sodas. For example, aspartame is converted to formaldehyde in the body. These toxins must be removed, or they can cause disease, kidney failure, malignancy, and various other painful problems.

This is not a situation that happens without any predictions; it is a dynamic problem and in the sense that it can be found as soon as it can be treated, change the diet, and it is possible what is causing the problem. You may still have partial kidney failure, as a rule. It takes a little time (or a completely terrible diet for a short period of time) to reach complete kidney failure. You would rather not have total kidney failure as this will require standard dialysis treatments to save your life.

Dialysis treatments explicitly cleanse the blood of wastes and toxins in the blood using a machine, taking into account the fact that your body can no longer be held responsible. Without treatment, you could die a very painful death. Kidney failure can be a consequence of long-term diabetes, hypertension, and unreliable diet, and can be the result of other health problems.

A kidney diet is related to the orientation of protein and phosphorus intake in your eating routine. It is also important to limit your sodium intake. By controlling these two variables, you can control the vast majority of toxins/wastes produced by your body and thus allow your kidney to function at 100%. If you do this early enough and really moderate your diets with extreme caution, you could prevent complete kidney failure. If you receive it early, you can fix it.

CPSIA information can be obtained
at www.ICGtesting.com
Printed in the USA
LVHW052122190221
679461LV00006B/707